Stroke of ~~Luck~~ Blessing

Chris Adkins

ISBN 978-1-63874-878-6 (paperback)
ISBN 978-1-63874-879-3 (digital)

Christian Faith Publishing, Inc.
832 Park Avenue
Meadville, PA 16335
www.christianfaithpublishing.com

Printed in the United States of America

Introduction

Blessing how? This story is my story, and one that you will see, as you continue to read, becomes a praise report for God. A story that the Lord Almighty has placed in my heart to share with as many people as I can. Every letter typed is for His glory and for Him alone. My journey to get to the point where I am is a winding one full of twists, turns, ups, and downs that turns into victory and restoration. A revival that caught me in the winds of faith taking me straight to him through every wind current I found myself in. I was heading up toward my heavenly Father, not understanding why.

If a survivor or caregiver is reading this, I pray this can help you! If not, you may find this miracle story a good read. I'm just a regular guy with a not-so-ordinary story. The process of the recovery of a stroke is different for us all. Reflection is a very important process that needs to take place to begin the healing of looking forward. Your attitude is a vital role on how you recover, along with being grateful you have been given this blessing to be alive.

In my case, the journey has been a long one. TIA, left cerebral stroke, right-frontal lobe stroke, and toss in locked-in syndrome—I was mad at the world and needed to get past my anger of even being in this position.

It is a blessing blocker to harbor anger and resentment. It is important that you not feel guilty that you feel this way. We are human and have emotion. Speaking of emotion, I believe I cried more after my strokes than my entire life. It's okay to do so, as we have a hard time controlling emotions—let alone a thought process.

If you have trouble even focusing due to recovery, in my case, a good dose of never-ending vertigo did not help. All this is a process to keep in perspective. I am blessed to have a wife that has stood (slept) by my side the entire way. The sixty-plus days I was in a hospital, the recovering, and the learning is exhausting. I was and am still a toddler with gray hair and a look in my eye that a toddler has—a look of learning something new, yet I had learned forty-five-plus years ago. I'm growing spiritually, leaps and bounds as I think you will see as you continue reading.

A Typical Day

Was not typical at all. I was in real estate, and the market was very strong. I had back-to-back appointments scheduled all day but felt it important to take my daughter to the doctor. I had no idea what lies ahead.

Picking up Kayley for the doctor appointment, I found myself at her appointment and began seeing things in a slanted way, feeling like I was seasick with no balance. After trying to go to the bathroom, I had to hold on to the wall and found a seat to sit in the waiting area.

Soon after my daughter came out to check on me, my left side of my face was drooping. I could not talk right and was drooling. Why is spit rolling out of the left side of my mouth? My tongue felt twisted, and I was scared. The security guard called an ambulance; it just so happened one was there, and I remember the staff saying a stroke trumps a baker act.

"Get him to a hospital!" and my nightmare began. My heart began to race so fast that it felt like I was having a heart attack. I didn't really even know what a stroke was, let alone the symptoms. I found myself looking at the EMT while on the stretcher, unable to communicate, knowing full-well this was bad, and knowing that this day was going to be a tough one.

I had never even ridden in an ambulance before. My first experience was as a child, only as an observer, when my aunt Carol was taken to the hospital for her fight with cancer, and the lights on the ambulance would take me back to the memory attached to my first experience of losing a loved one. Now here I am, in an ambulance and not knowing what to do.

Anxiety began to fill my head with questions. Where am I going? They are telling me it's a stroke. What is that? Why do I feel seasick? Where is my daughter, Kayley? Gosh, I'm glad I wasn't driving when this happened. Has anyone called my wife? My mind was racing, as you can imagine, I'm sure.

In my mind, I was thinking, *I wonder if I can still make my three-o'clock appointment I had that day with a client.*

The ambulance driver would say, "You're going to be okay, bud." The EMT guy in back with me was trying to keep me calm, and I was just looking up at the ceiling, not even giving a thought to pray about my situation. I thought I could handle whatever came my way.

Looking back, I gotta say, *Wow, I thought I was something.* I was a powerlifter and forty-nine years old, bench pressing over five hundred pounds with ease. How am I in this position after hearing my ambulance driver tell me I was having a stroke? I thought, once at the hospital, I would be taken care of.

If anyone reading this has a loved one in the hospital, be a voice for him or her. I pray you get a doctor that knows what they're doing and spends every second trying to help you and not judging. I was always under the impression that doctors are not to be questioned: they know what they're doing. After all the schooling they have had, they are good at what they do. Wrong—they are still human and make mistakes.

I pray for you to stand up if something doesn't feel right, ask them questions, and stand up for your loved ones. Be their voice. If a tele doc is used, ask them, "Why am I not talking to a live doctor here?" Tele doc is used when there are not enough doctors. I was unfortunately there on a Friday afternoon and at the end of the month. Season in my area is from January to Easter, and that is when people vacation and a lot of the working folks in the area take three-day weekend. With days in the '80s, why not?

I'm not encouraging you to be rude or disrespectful at all: just ask questions, and do your own research. As vertigo kicked in stronger than ever, the doctor on call could not get past my size and physique's stature. My wife and kids showed up, and I was told my oldest—my son—was on his way from Tampa and would be here soon. My poor wife was trying to talk to me, and I could not stop dry heaving and asked her to move to my right side, as my left eye was twitching so badly I could not see out of it.

I found myself getting very upset that it was taking so long to figure this out when the guys in the ambulance said it was a stroke. I could see something on my left side that looked like a box on the wall. There were many people in that room that day, and I was told, "That's a $50,000 shot, and it looks like you won't need it." (This is a TPA, or commonly referred to as a clot buster.) I was lucky they saved me the money.

Luck and money are two words that are not reassuring in a hospital; maybe Vegas, but not here. While still having all these symptoms, plus having gotten to the hospital in thirteen minutes, I was like, *Whatever, JUST FIX IT.* I'm not sure how much time was spent talking about my size, steroid use, and that it was seizures, but it was a long time. Therefore, not convinced it was a stroke.

After accusing me of steroid use (it's called years of work), tests were run; and before I knew it, I was in a hospital room. Once in the room, I remember being hooked up to so many IVs in my arm (later I would be told eleven). Now being treated for meningitis, my kidneys were beginning to shut down. I was in a nightmare and just wanted it to be over. All the while, my head was pounding, and I could feel my eyes beginning to pop out of my skull. And I kept trying to rub my eyes, thinking blood was coming out. I now had slurred speech so bad that I could not communicate.

I remember cold dots on my face as they were trying to see if I would have a seizure, still thinking it wasn't a stroke and believing it was a seizure. Lying in bed, I was so confused why I was not feeling the pressure being released and continued to build my headache. Now was the worst I can ever remember; something was different about this—not a take-an-aspirin kind of headache, but one that I had never felt before. Felt like the top of my head was going to blow off.

One thing led to another, as I was already close to death. I kept asking myself, "So this is how it ends?" I did not see this coming, obviously. It was as if the perfect storm were brewing, and what could go wrong was. I felt really sad that I would not get to say my good-byes to my wife, kids, and family members. It makes you think how fast life can change.

The one thing that did happen is clarity that I was screwed! March 31, 2016, would be my last day of living a normal life, but the start of a new way of living. I was a believer before all this, but I would call myself a babe in the woods when it came to my spiritual walk.

I was a regular church attender and knew of God, but not near the depths I was about to experience. I was one that thought I knew him and thought I did have a relationship. One that treats him like a genie in a bottle. Asking for what I want, then when finished, put him back until I need him again. What I had was one based on my convenience. I would seek prayer on my time. If it was a good time for me, I would be okay with praying.

I was in control of my life, and if I had the time for God, then I would talk to him. Talk to him with a hidden agenda of asking for what I wanted. Gone would be the days of dressing myself, going to the bathroom, walking, taking showers, being unable to close my eyes while washing my hair, fishing, playing basketball, throwing a football with my son during football season, and even sleeping like I used to—just to name a few. Things that we take for granted every day are a struggle for the disabled person.

A brain injury is one that people don't see visually from the out-side, but it effects *all* of you and all your loved ones. The brain is the central control tower, and it sends messages to your body for all func-tion. If a control tower were shut down at an airport, all flights in and out would be canceled. When the brain shuts down or is injured, then nothing works. There is no direction. You may think a thought or a movement, but unless the brain communicates it, there will be nothing. Having a brain injury of any kind is a real game changer; you no longer can function the way you use to. It is a helpless feeling that lingers deep within us that, if we let it, will control us.

Being the central control tower, it wants to shut down to avoid anymore pain, like you would stop all flights. To move forward, I find it helpful to look for what I call "little victories." An example: this morning for me was noticing one of my pre-tied shoes was untied. I picked my shoe up and tied my shoe the best I could then placed it on my foot. That's a little victory.

I did not have my morning pee, so I may have peed my shorts—we will call it a draw morning so far, but I still am excited about my shoe being tied though. Misty may not be excited about the urine smell in the hamper, but we will rejoice about the shoe tying.

Another example: yesterday I got the mail by myself—granted, it's right by the front door—but to me that's a little victory because I knew which key it was, opened the front door, stepped down a step, opened the mailbox, got the mail, and brought it inside and laid it on the table. That's a multiple thought process for me, and I feel pretty darn good about it.

Funny how no matter what age we are, a little praise goes a long way. My wife was there to witness this, and I must admit my chest began to puff with pride. To most people they would read this and say, "That's not that hard to do" or "It's sad that this seems like a big deal." This is where attitude of gratitude comes in to play. We can control how we respond to a challenge. We laugh a lot at some of the things I do. It's amusing to think that some of my reactions are so childlike. I have so many examples of this.

I have to be told many times how to do things and still forget. Typing this book is one that is fresh in my mind. The one finger typing and trying to figure out how to hold the cap button down with my left finger is comical. I have typed a ton of the letter *A*, only to have to go back and correct it many times, causing this to turn into a multitude of excruciating time to get my story complete.

There has been a lot of twelve-hour-plus days to only get a few pages completed. It's funny to me, and another example of perseverance I hope will become part of my legacy I leave behind.

I have been blessed with a never-quit attitude that was in me at an early age from my father telling and, more importantly, showing me every single day without fail. You can't stop anyone from achieving anything if they simply don't quit. That's a whole different topic or even book I could write. If I start now, it could be released as early as 2025. I want to list a few facts I looked up on the American Stroke Association website I want to share with you.

Fact

A few stroke facts:

- Someone in the US has a stoke every forty seconds.
- Every four minutes, someone dies of stroke.
- Over 795,000 people in the US alone has a stoke annually.
- 87% of strokes are ischemic.
- 40% of stroke survivors are depressed, per the American Stroke Association.
- FAST: F—Face drooping, A—Arm weakening, S—Speech slurred, T—Time to call 911.
- Luke Perry, Bill Paxton, Richard Nixon, Cary Grant, John Singleton, Rue McClanahan, Aaron Spelling, Winston Churchill, Isaac Hayes, Clarence Clemons, Rick James— just to name a few we have lost to stroke. If you are a stroke survivor and you reading this, you are a miracle, and I am so proud of you.

Chip the Chipster

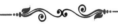

I wanted to dedicate a part of my book to Chip who, after watching the videos, is a big reason why I was able to start my PT quickly. He would push me every day; he could tell that I was determined and wanted to do the work necessary to improve my actions would show as I still could not speak. From the looks of the video material, just trying to sit up after lying in bed for almost a month was tough, then to try and move my legs was hard to watch.

It took me back to right where this was happening and not being able to speak but hear words of encouragement from Chip and my wife to keep on keeping on. I can see from the videos the time delay it would take me to communicate from my brain to my legs for movement. The concentration in my eyes to get movement says it all—sometimes no movement at all is heartbreaking to see.

As I began to progress a little by May 7, I could sit in a wheelchair and attempt to stand up. By the following week, I was using a bike to peddle while holding on to handles so I wouldn't fall over. I would celebrate my fiftieth birthday on the seventeenth at a place called Brookdale to take it to the next level. Many family members, friends, and staff would be there to celebrate.

I can remember eating the birthday cake as if I had not eaten in a long time. It tasted like a slice or slices, in my case, of heaven and was made with love. My left leg was still not confident enough to put weight on it, so that was the main focus. My right was taking a pounding. Trying to get your brain to even remember that I have a left side at all is, in itself, a daily task to this day. I sometimes still catch myself trying to function with just my right side.

Anyone reading this as a survivor: please don't give up. We are here, and let's try to make the best of what we have, whatever that may be...

Faith, Hope, and Love

These are three words that are powerful to me. *Faith* is complete trust or confidence in someone or something, and *hope* is a feeling of expectation and desire for a certain thing. *Love* is an intense feeling of deep affection. Notice that all three of these explains God and His love for us.

> And now these three remain: faith, hope, and love. But the greatest is love. (1 Corinthians 13:13)

This scripture pretty much sums it up. Having these words to hang on to during times of trial will help anyone to come through the valley. The valley is a place we all have to go through to get to that mountain and be able to look back over the valley to see what you walked through.

Being driven to mountaintops has become a favorite of mine to do, reflecting on the valley in a deep, spiritual way. We moved to West US for the solitude and to live with the rest of my life on disability. It didn't take us long to figure out that Southwest Florida was now out of our reach and simply could not be afforded anymore. We left a lot of family behind to do it but had prayed diligently over the move.

> Faith is confidence in what we hope for and assurance about what we do not see. (Hebrews 11:1)

This is my life verse and what I held on to while in my coma.

As a believer, I felt I could make it through. Notice I said, "Looking back, I actually thought that I could do anything with God by my side." While in a battle to survive, God showed me that I (me) cannot do anything without Him! For without Him, I am nothing. We actually think we can do things on our own. I would like to save you a lot of time and thought on this subject. We are nothing without Him!

While in my coma, I faced what I recall was the black hole of hell! It was moving like it was a tornado of fire—only it was in reverse, as it was rotating in a downward spiral. With each turn, it revealed souls that were screaming for me to get them out. Faces, arms, and legs flailing with each turn. It had a smell like a musty old bard to me.

Looking at this, it was scary and made me feel like a child wanting protection. What was I to do? It was me; it was me that was looking in and living the horror that had a hold of me. I literally was in the most horrific movie I had ever seen, let alone actually be the main character that wanted no part of this movie.

With each turn of the twister of death, I could see so many people that were in hell. The bottom of the twister was a blazing fire that was the last stop for these souls. Reaching for anything they could to get out before reaching the bottom, I knew the only way out was Jesus. I still had a choice. Their souls would be in eternal hell forever. There were so many that I would watch this circular pit with each turn. I swear I think I would see more each time it turned.

I found myself actually feeling hot. Later I would be told I had a fever of 104 for some time. The longer I stood at the edge of the twister looking down, Satan was looking to push me in, yet I was not going!

Then he decided to take me to a room down a dark hallway where I would see body parts on the floor; the amount of blood that was there made me gag. I was then tied down on a large table saw that looked like it was just used with flesh and bone all over it. I could hear the saw being turned on and coming toward me. It felt like an eternity before the blades were cutting through my flesh.

Part of my feeling of the heat had to be the urine all over me, trembling with so much fear yet not giving in to this. The first thing that was sawed off was my left arm. I could hear the metal hitting my bone and pieces of my flesh and bones all over me. I was not going to give in and was not going to give Satan any satisfaction in doing this.

I knew a powerful God—that is, my Father—and started to scream at the top of my lungs, "I LOVE YOU, GOD." I did not scream for help, because I strangely had a peace that if this is how it goes down, then so be it.

The left leg was cut off, and He showed up. I have read about dreams of amputation and the common theme is sacrifice and loss of control. The sacrifice for me was giving it all to God at any cost. If He gave His only begotten son then to me, I had no room to complain about the situation I was in. It was so real that it was real if that makes any sense.

The meaning of *sacrifice*, as written in the dictionary, is "surrendering a possession as an offering to God as an act of slaughter, an animal or person; a loss for the sake of a better cause."

In the situation I was in, I really didn't care about the outcome; I did care that my love for Him is more than anything the enemy could throw at me, or in my case, saw off me. It's at that moment when you talk the talk or walk the walk. I would not waiver, and I believe God knew it and rewarded me by literally taking it from that point on and giving me the courage to see this journey through to the end.

I am so happy to share this because I pray that others, when faced with any kind of adversity in life, sacrifice for the goodness of God. As for the loss of control, here comes that part of the one hundred percent I was holding back, actually thinking I even had control. Remember earlier on I thought I was the man and I could handle anything thrown at me? This is where the big slice of humble pie comes in. In my case, a whole humble pie.

I really thought, in my mind, that I could do all things with me at the wheel. God is not the passenger here; He sees the beginning and the end, even knowing what we are going to do before we do it. He knew that while in my many MRI scans.

When asked what song I wanted to hear, it would be Tim McGraw's "Humble and Kind." I consider myself kind, but humble was an area of improvement for me. I now find it amusing that we think we have any control—*wrong*. The number here is zero. Us humans want the easy way out; this is just how we are wired. Teaching our minds to be strong should be a part of our training daily. With God's grace, we can do all through him. God is in control but does not take control. He is with us, and the closer we get to Him, the quicker we can discern, therefore affecting our judgement.

Soon after repeating "Show Me Your Glory" by third day, this seemed to speed up the process; and before I knew it, my left leg was severed. I shouted Hebrews 11:1, "Faith is being sure of what we hope for and certain of what we do not see." I knew my God and Savior would protect me.

As I turn my head to the left to see half my body gone, tears rolling down my face, I saw Misty, and I whispered, "Go under the table." I wanted her to hide from this and not see what was happening to me as my head was turned to the left and my right leg was cut off. Hoping, with every last breath, that the devil would not see her. I didn't know it yet, but soon my eyes would be gouged out and I was in the dark. Now I had no way of knowing what was next. I had a dream later that I was given eyes from a dog. Strange, I know, but at the time, I was in this dream/nightmare.

At that moment, I was shown the gates of heaven. What a beautiful sight these eyes have seen. I became so comfortable and at peace. I really didn't care what Satan was going to do to me. I remember saying in my mind, *Bring it on! I'm going to heaven!*

God revealed Himself and said, "I have got it from here. I'm not finished with you yet, son". I was so happy when He showed His face. In the blink of an eye, all darkness turned to light, the brightest light I had ever seen—almost a blinding light, yet a light that was one of protection and total peace.

I will never forget the love He's shown me and continues to show me every day. As for me and my house, we will serve the Lord resonates. I'm literally coming out swinging—not in a physical sense, but one of a mission to show God's love everywhere I go. If what I say offends anyone, then so be it. Not only did God tell me to spread His love, but He showed me.

Gratitude is overflowing in me so much so that I have been approached by people asking, "Why are you so happy?" or "What is different about you?" Quite a few of my friends I had before my strokes have faded away for whatever reason. I will say this: the ones that are still here, our relationship has gotten stronger and on a much more personal level. I leave no doubt where I stand, and if you're not with me, then get out of my way. I'm on a mission and have learned that I won't waste any time on something that my Lord and savior doesn't call me to pursue.

If God is for us, who can be against us?
(Romans 8:31)

Time is our most valuable asset we have on Earth, so make the most of it and be the best at whatever it is you do. I sound like a motivational speaker sometimes. I'm motivated by my faith and hope that you are too. Speaking of hope, to me, hope is very powerful. I have hope that any survivors or caregivers out there have hope; if not, let's find it together. I have hope every day that I will be given an opportunity to spread it.

Once you choose hope, anything's possible.
(Christopher Reeve)

I was told that I would have a life like him as my best case in the future. I had hope like Christopher, and by the grace of God, I am able to function with my disabilities.

I was going to be as much like God as I could and bring as many people to him. Knowing how bad hell is, I want no one to go there, and it actually scares me to even write about it. I know fear is not of the Lord; but I got to tell you, in this case, I was so scared. I now have to surround myself with scripture to feel protected.

The thing is, that the enemy will find any way he can to get in your head and cause doubt, knowing our every weakness. Why do you think there are so many people with drug and alcohol addictions? This is what he wants: to destroy you and keep you from team Jesus adding another member.

As the crack of doubt widens, so does the feeling of wanting to numb the pain. The downward spiral starts, and the short-term fix leads to a blessing blocker in our lives. You are a child of the Most High God, and you are special to him. Let me ask you this: in a typical day for you, how much time do you spend getting to know Him? My answer pre-stroke was little. I start every day now, reading scripture, and I'm on the second time reading the Bible cover-to-cover. What time you put into something is what you get out of it. A relationship needs nurturing and is not a relationship at all when it's one-sided.

As I write this, I'm sure some of you may not like my story. Then I'm sorry it wasn't meant for you. Someone will find this as a wake-up call and find the Lord, or shall I say, seek Him. If one person reads this and becomes a follower of Christ, then this was a success. As a stroke and locked-in survivor, this has been very difficult for me to write. Many hours and many times talking in circles; I apologize if, at times, this is hard to follow.

As you can see from the cover of my book, I don't have much to work with. Literally almost half of my brain is a black mass. I have been told that I will never have the use of that space again, yet somehow my brain is rewiring itself. I know what that somehow is and find it a miracle that I can do the things I can do today. We joke around our home that I'm a half-brain, yet there's not much difference in the brain power I had before March 31, 2016. I find life so different now because my thoughts take so much time to communicate, let alone write them down.

The enemy was putting doubt in my mind and cutting off my limbs—yes, *limbs*. I tolerated the pain for awhile, all the while on fire. My wife said my fever would spike while in my coma. I had a 104-degree fever for some time. Not until I said, "I can't do this, God" did He show me His face and said, *I have it from here.* I was entering heaven and literally could see my resting place. God told me He is not finished with me, and I woke up from my coma.

The flesh side of us thinks we can do things on our terms. We go down the path we think is the correct one and soon realize that we are headed the wrong way. Stubborn people, myself included, just try another path; and before you know, it we have taken so many wrong paths that we are just living life going in circles, thinking we will figure this out when all we had to do was seek God first.

Nothing is possible without Him, and the sooner we realize this, the less time we will waste on taking the wrong path. He sees us doing this, and I can only imagine how He must find us amusing. He does have a sense of humor: look at the platypus (one crazy-looking creature that is a mammal that lays eggs). I find myself reflecting on how we send out prayers when things are tough and go to Him as a last resort, when we should go to Him first. As for me, He is my best friend who knows everything about me, including all my weaknesses (and it is a long list). I am blessed to be where I am to have a relationship of this kind.

He is one of a kind, obviously. He certainly lets me know when I am in the flesh; it happens to all of us—the more we try to be like him, the quicker we realize we are of the flesh and respond according to our faith. The tongue is just vicious. My first marriage was one that I had to protect my kids and myself, so I always had a few choice words in the chamber, so to speak. I'm not proud of who I was then, but I always protected my children the best I could. And yet he encourages me when I stand strong in faith: slow to speak, slow to anger.

> Know this, my beloved brothers: let every person be quick to hear, slow to speak, slow to anger; for the anger of man does not produce the righteousness of God. Therefore, put away all filthiness and rampant wickedness and receive with meekness the implanted word, which is able to save your souls. But be doers of the world, and not hearers only, deceiving yourselves. For if anyone is a hearer of the world and not a doer, he is

like a man who looks intently at his natural face
in a mirror. (James 1:19–27)

Faith is being sure of what we hope for and
certain of what we do not see. Without faith, it is
impossible to please God. (Hebrews 11:1)

I mention this again for a reason. When you think of a brain
injury, you cannot see it, but a survivor must face that which you
may not see. But our faith is what has gotten us this far and will continue to keep us going! Ask yourself, How can I bless someone today?
Genuine interest in them is so important.

When God pricks your heart, then do it! No matter what you
think, God knows what's best. I find that if we just make the intro-
duction and let God use us as a vessel, He will take care of the rest.
You are a child of God, and He is so proud of you for obeying Him.

Love is the universal language that we all understand. Think
about it: no matter what country you see—while watching, say, a
documentary—love can be felt in any language. God is love. My kids
attended a Christian school and had a teacher that would say "Agape
love," referring to *unconditional love*—the love of God for man and
of man for God. This was exciting for the kids to share with me. I
honestly hadn't a clue what it meant but soon understood thanks to
them.

*****

There is a big difference in the kind of strokes. TIA is a transient
ischemic attack stroke, which really is a big warning sign of stroke
is coming. If treated, the so-called ministroke can be treated at 6:00
a.m. to noon, or at the highest number of TIA; mine was at 1:00
p.m. One in three people having a TIA will have a stroke within a
year.

Ischemic stroke (which, in my case, was my second stroke).
Eighty-seven percent of strokes are ischemic. I then had a hemor-
rhagic stroke after a spinal tap that put me in a coma. This is the

part where it gets a little scary. I was not given what is called a TPA or clot buster.

My doctor was still stuck on me being a steroid-taking bodybuilder who did not fit the profile at forty-nine, sticking to that theory along with seizures being my health challenge. I never took steroids and had never had a seizure before.

It's tough when in your mind you know it's a stroke while vomiting and left-eye twitching. You cannot speak, all the while replaying in my mind the ambulance, and the paramedics telling me I'm having a stroke and will be okay. The rest of my journey is one of survival, faith, and nothing short of a miracle. This is one heck of a ride, so I hope this helps someone out there.

I write this out of a promise I made to God that I will share this miracle with as many as I can. As I finish this book, it will be my five-year "stroke-versary." And as I continue writing, I just received a call from my aunt Lois that my uncle Lyndon is having a TIA and is in the ER. The power of prayer is at work, and we pray that he gets a doctor that is informed in the area of stroke; and time is vital.

My aunt remembered the FAST acronym, and he had all of the signs; so the T in FAST was the last step (meaning time), and he got there quickly. (Praise God.) My heart is so troubled right now; this is just the beginning of the fight of his life. He is a pastor in Eastern Kentucky, and we all know where he is going. It's in God's hands as to when he goes. We pray for his wife and kids and all the family to be an anchor in this storm.

As I said earlier, go head into the storm! It took me a long time to write this, and a lot of emotions came flooding back—like a dam had broken in my soul, starting with a crack and busting wide open with a ton of emotions. Now as I type away, the emotions are raw again, knowing I have a loved one in the fight like I was. This is just another example that we all are at risk anytime, and there are no age restrictions to this movie.

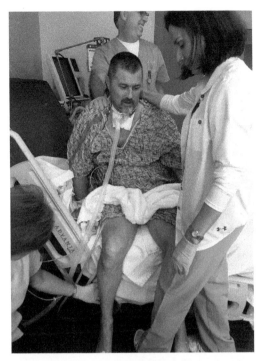

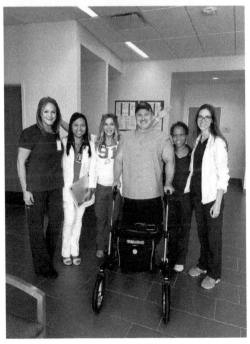

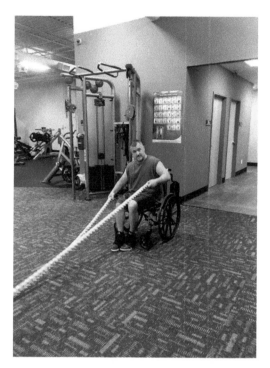

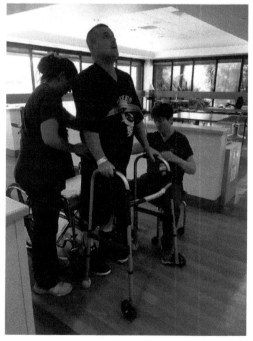

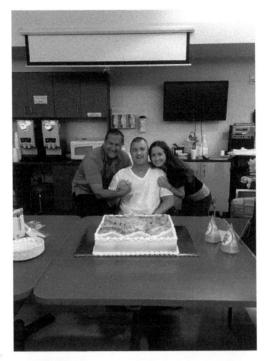

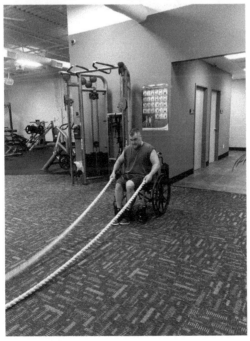

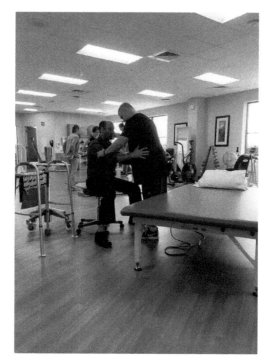

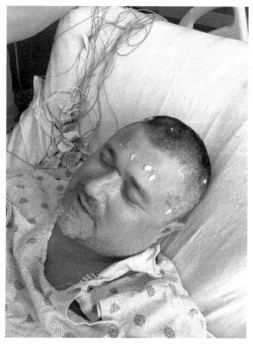

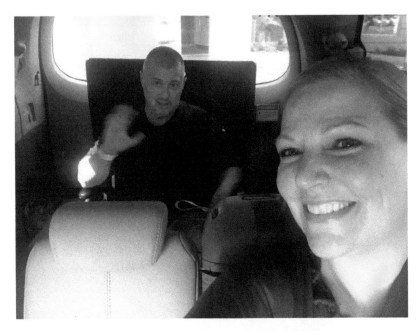

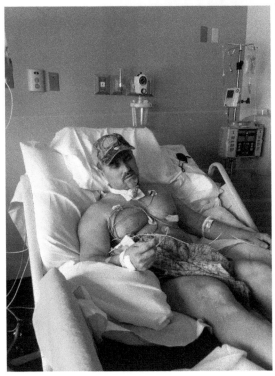

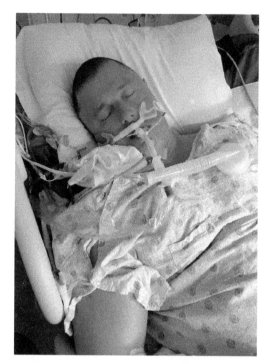

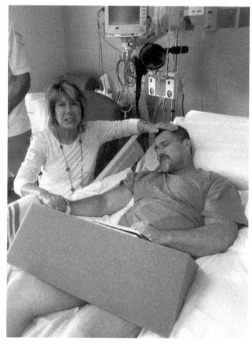

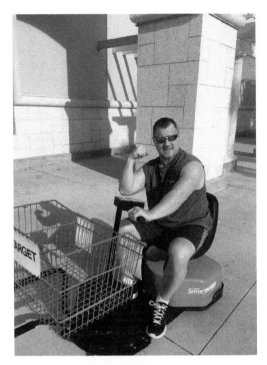

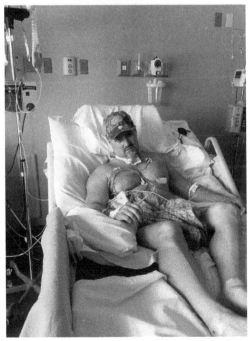

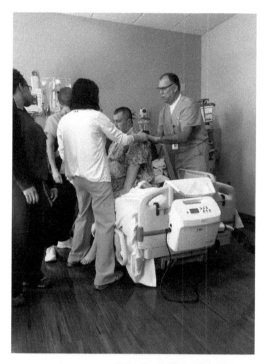

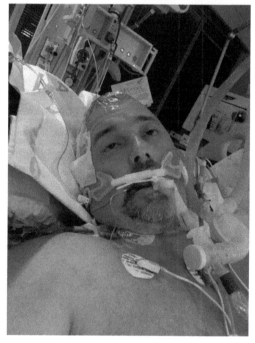

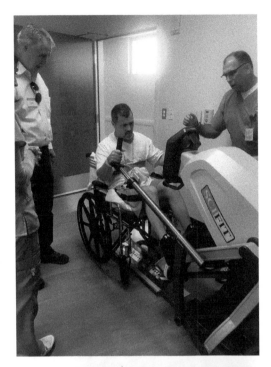

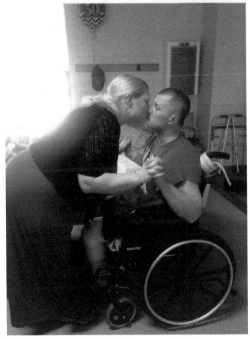

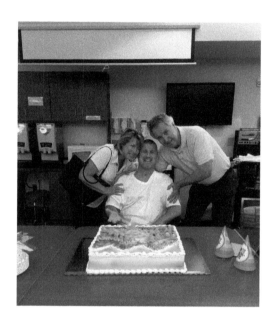

History Background

I named my left side Lefty to talk to it and try and get my arm or leg to follow. Muscle memory would have to kick in at some point. Reflecting back, there are factors that saved me—God, wife, support, and my weight lifting had paid off.

Going back eight years prior to my first stroke, I began lifting weight at age forty-one with my son. I was going through an awful divorce, and I needed an out. After defeating alcohol years before, I was not going back there! So a 178-pound forty-one-year-old man was going to commit to going to the gym as often as possible. Six days a week—at least an hour a day—and eight years later, I weighed 245 pounds and was solid muscle.

I had many people that helped me to achieve this. Jabz would become my second home, putting all I had into becoming a power lifter. I quickly was lifting all the weight on the machines and went to free weights; the bench was my favorite. I have short arms, so less distance to push. I did break six hundred pounds and really was on my way to breaking records for my age group nationally. I would have to say this helped me to survive and have a grasp of what I would have to do to learn things over again! They ran many tests and could never find what caused my strokes. I was a miracle that drove the science part of this crazy.

After going through many blood tests, they would all come back with the same results of "we don't know why." I wanted to get to PT as fast as possible, so Chip and I—along with my wife and great nurses—were off to PT as often as I could take it. I found myself so focused on PT that I was doing all this and was not able to talk, so speech therapy and OT had to be a part of it as well. Trouble is—as a stroke survivor—four weeks from having them, I was tired. It seemed I would push as hard as I could every day and rest to be able to progress.

Almost five years later, I am doing the same thing. I want to get better and dream of walking someday. Just to be able to walk unassisted and without having to look down at every step. I think it's important to never give up on what your dreams are. No one has walked in your shoes as a survivor, nor do I want anyone to go through what I went through and continue to go through daily.

Fighting as desperately as a person can a vicious battle to not let the enemy steal my joy, filling my head with doubt. Fighting to breathe the heat off my body, every muscle trying to grasp what is happening and slowly losing control over my body. Imagine you cannot tell your body to do anything you wanted to do; there is a way of feeling the positive energy I could feel—positive and also negative. I would shut down when I would hear negative thoughts, trying not to let them in my space. I find comfort in dealing with what's in front of me and not looking back.

The gym became my sanctuary again. This is where I knew I could get on a faster track to recovery. I was released in early June and went right to work. First challenge: going home to a two-story house with a master bedroom upstairs. My wife would have to wheel me from the car to the front door with steps along the way; we knew we were in trouble. This was going to be a bigger challenge than we expected.

Learning how to get out of the wheelchair was tough. I still had a hard time with balance and tinnitus—this constant ringing (in my case, my left ear). Trying not to get frustrated at yourself is tough. I kept repeating, "God is in control. He got me this far. I have a responsibility to glorify Him," and all I'm doing now is getting out of the wheelchair.

*****

What do I do now? There's no shower downstairs; it's in the master bedroom upstairs. There were sixteen steps to get to the master bedroom up there. I simply cannot do this for a month or so without complete exhaustion. We decided we would get a bed in the dining room downstairs.

We then had to think about me taking a shower. The gym had a shower that was ADA-accessible. Misty would take me to the gym so I could begin training and help me to take a shower. Not being able to get out of the wheelchair, Misty would have to help me and place my hands on the grab bars, all the while feeling like I was standing on ice. I cannot even raise a dumbbell, let alone get out of my wheelchair, so I would have her help me to get on a machine. The highlight of my day was going to the gym…

I used ropes as part of my training. I could not lift the ropes at all, so I asked my wife to take out the side panels of the wheelchair. I knew the motion but could not get movement. I remember telling myself, "I have to do this for God and be an example of what pure determination looks like." I slowly began to move my right arm and noticed that Lefty was curious and began to show interest. Lefty moved!

Before I knew it, I was moving both arms while holding the ropes. It was nothing fancy by any means, but I was doing it and was so excited to show the kids. My son would go with me to the gym to help encourage me. This became my passion to grind it out every day. My poor wife, Misty, was my chaperone, driving me to the gym, PT and doctor appointments, and home—plus, running the newly adapted ADA household was to become her new normal.

My new normal was attacking everything with more determination than I had ever before. I wanted to break records in all my PT and OT appointments. I always tried my best every day. (It's important to remember we all have bad days.) I had no idea that all I learned would be gone when I woke in the morning. My brain is slow-moving in the morning. I really just wanted to roll over and go back to sleep. Finding a balance for the proper rest takes time and a lot of trial and error. You will begin to know how hard you can push yourself and rest as well—it's a fine line that can't be flirted with that often, so keep that in mind.

Being a caregiver is a difficult thing to do and, unfortunately, is sometimes not appreciated enough. The mood swings are normal, or so I have been told. I find quiet time with the Lord—my peace to carry on and show love and thankfulness for the help I have and continue to receive.

Looking back, there were times I was difficult, to say the least. It's beyond humbling when you can't control your bowels, tie your shoes, put clothes on, or even just general hygiene. The caregiver is always there and knows your every move. Many times Misty would ask if I did a pooh-pooh poopy. I adamantly denied it like a toddler, and sure enough, she would check my shorts and there was a poopy indeed. When driving me anywhere, I would have a pee cup with me and had a fifty-fifty shot at best of hitting the cup. There were many peed-on shorts and shirts. I would always say, "So what!" It was just the new me, and this was how it was going to be.

When I was younger, I never understood, while talking with customers, how I would be talking with them and they would be letting air. I learned to just ignore and continue talking. Well I'm that guy now. This may be a little off topic, but I want all the loved ones out there to know that! Living with a survivor to know that this is just us, and what you see is what you get. It's as if the filter we had as adults reverts back to childhood; hard to explain, but the love we have for you all hasn't changed a bit. In fact, I would bet that most survivors you ask would say it actually has gotten deeper, only harder to communicate sometimes. I started a new thing a few years back: every morning, I make Misty coffee and put it in a styrofoam cup so I can draw a heart on it. This takes me time to do it; but it's a big deal to me, so I get excited when I complete it. Not the prettiest of things, but I try…

The amount of effort it takes for me to get ready on a daily basis takes a toll. Just to function is exhausting for me. The aftereffects of which is a long list, starting from the obvious: head, thoughts, etc.; tinnitus; loss of hearing in left ear; exhaustion; twitching in my left eye when I open it; hernia from pick line; balance to even try and stand circulation in my legs; foot drop on right side; left foot's toe is lifted up so I wear out shoes that are cloth material; and vertigo quite often. All this and I have to start over again every morning all the while repeating God is greater than all this!

I find that a part of my brain that cared, now doesn't. In fact, I don't sweat the small stuff anymore, down to my clothes matching; some of my outfits are quite eye-catching. If Misty did not switch out my clothes, I would wear the same shorts and cut-off shirt every day! (My Popeye shirt with the sleeves cut out is my fave.) It helps me to lie in bed when I wake to think through what I need to do and the energy it will take to do them.

I sleep on the left side of the bed so I can turn my dominant right leg to get out of bed. I place my pre-tied shoes together at the foot of the bed and begin my walk to the bathroom. I say all this because from this point on, I have to think if I have the energy to take a morning shower. Most of the time I don't; instead I find evening showers are a little easier on me.

Mornings bring a slow start. Brushing my teeth, shave, and add a BM, and I'm good for forty-five minutes. I take seven different meds in the morning, and I like to do this on my own (Misty is always close by to check). I am a toddler at times and may come out to the breakfast table with no underwear on, shaving lotion still on my face, and to add to the handsomeness, toothpaste all over my face.

I simply can't resist trying to kiss my wife in the morning to see what kind of response I get. I am blessed, so most of the time she just goes along with it. Gym shorts and sleeveless shirts seem to be my go-to every day. A brain injury is difficult to explain, yet one that people can't see.

I have many examples of being judged on how I look. I still look like a muscle head so many times. I'm asked, "What is wrong with you? Do you really need a disabled sticker on your car?" Sometimes the emotion of the situation can really get to me. I never imagined I would be put in a position to have to try and explain that I'm disabled. I chose to wear a knee brace so visually it looked like I had something wrong with me. I found this worked wonders for us going out in public. Putting a knee brace on is part of my everyday ritual now. I can quickly discern sincerity and decide if I'm going to just go with the knee injury or take the time time to give a short version of my story. God leads me on this and I obey. The flesh is a real challenge for all of us-I still ask him do I really have to walk up to this stranger? Who am I to even question it!. I will say this, every time I do as he says I walk away being blessed myself. God wants us to stretch our faith every day-we have many times given every dollar we had left to a homeless person, not out of pity but out of love and kindness to others just because we have a dark past the forgiveness you get when becoming a team Jesus member is a chance to be a light in this dark world. People will disappoint and Jesus never fails us. Why is it so hard for us to grasp this?

Activity for Recovery

Strive for forty-five seconds now and then; what I mean by this is I see so many people in the gym that would rather lift what I call "nickels, dimes, and quarters," never really pushing themselves to the forty-five plates. Just when you think you cannot do another rep or finish an exercise, you have one more in you. Muhammad Ali was once asked, "How many push ups can you do?"

His response, "I don't know. I don't start counting until it hurts." And there you go: his record speaks for itself. At twelve years old, his bike was stolen, and he decided he was going to learn to box—the rest is history. My question is, If you're afraid to try when you are healthy, what will you do in a trial?

Every stroke is different, and every recovery is as well. This means a big part is in your hands. Go at your own pace. Keep moving forward. A little progress can go a long way. Try lying on a bed and stretching arms out, like making a snow angel. Begin lifting both affected and unaffected arms and legs together. Any movement is moving. This took me a week to get my movement at all.

The first two days in a row, nothing happened, and I had to take an hour nap after attempting. My first exercise was sitting up; this took me only ten seconds to sit up before I needed to lie back down, and that was with the help of four hospital staff to assist moving me. At home, I would use knee pads to crawl to the kitchen sink to grab the lip of the sink to pull myself up. Once up, I figured, *While here, I will attempt a squat action to get my left leg to follow.*

After many failed attempts, I began to be able to do it! We had an island in the kitchen, and I would always visualize myself being able to walk around it while holding on to the bar area. I can remember, as if it were yesterday, how exhausted I was doing this. It was a grand total of eleven steps to do this. I would make this a daily routine whether I wanted to or not. Now I find myself thinking of a routine: stretches on the bed, walk to kitchen (not crawl) or use my four-pronged cane to get there, go to the sink and do squats, walk around the island of the kitchen and land on a chair in the great room. Piece of cake.

Wrong. I had bitten off more than I could chew and would ask for help to get back to bed. While falling asleep, dreaming of some-day soon being able to complete the routine, I found that I was never satisfied with my progress. Happy I was making progress, I wanted to do more all the time! I sound a little off my rocker sometimes; I guess because I am different in many ways. Having been told I would never even get out of a wheelchair was always playing over and over in my mind. I don't think I would be where I am today if I didn't push myself every day a little harder and praise Him every step of the way.

*****

Fast forward to Thanksgiving 2016, and I completed a 5k (called the turkey trot) in a mind blowing one hour—yes, one hour. Surprise: I was the last one to finish. This was hard for me, as in my past, I was a competitive runner that could easily finish in under sixteen minutes. Most runners complete it in eight- to ten-minute miles. I still go back to my running days and long to hear the wind as I run, feeling like floating.

My kids, nephew, and my biggest fan, my wife, walked with me. I used my walker and wore out the top of my left shoe in walking this. My left toe was exposed through the mesh of my shoe. The staff that had organized the race made sure the last runner is always in. It was me, and it was nice to hear cheers as I crossed the finish line. No sooner had I finished and taken a few pictures that I was thinking of the next 5k and doing it in under an hour.

I set my sights on a run that our church was sponsoring in July (yes, I said July) in south Florida. I had a crew with me this time as well: my sister and her husband, Rhett, walked with us. It was a brutally hot day that was not going to stop me. I was at the starting line with bottled water in the basket of my walker, and I was off. Quickly we settled into being the last ones in the race. I was okay with this, as my goal was clearly to better my last race time. It is better for me when I don't have to worry about other runners running into me. I could easily fall over, and I can hear timber in the back of my mind.

When I walk anywhere, I have to look for grass in case I have to fall. We found ourselves in a moment of truth as the summer sun started to heat the asphalt and heat began to rise off it that I needed to somehow pick up the pace. Balance is one of the hardest things for me to handle, so I have to look down and am unable to look straight away. I began to count off my steps. Once I got to 1,227 steps, I could see the finish line; or shall I say, my crew told me I was close. We had picked up two members of our church along the way. I finished in fifty-six minutes. Not an ESPN top ten by any means, but I did what I set out to do.

*****

What plans do we have? Plans don't always work out. I have a new way of looking at plans: seek God's advice first—most men and some women I'm sure just keep focused on what the plan is. Did God have the same plan? When you get punched in the gut, you are taken back and start asking, "Why is this not working?" Let's review: did you ask God? In my case, I found myself saying, "I give it all to you, Lord," but holding back a good ten percent just in case I could pull this off myself.

Looking back now, what an idiot I was. I actually realized while in my coma, battling to stay alive, I was not a hundred percent on giving it to God (stubborn mule). This attitude is playing right into the devil's hand. Once I finally said, "Lord, I am ready to go to heaven. It is up to you." I figured it was a win-win situation for me: heaven or earth.

He answered and told me, *I'm not finished with you yet, son!* I woke up from my coma to only have locked-in syndrome as well.

Locked-in syndrome is basically when you are locked in your body, unable to move anything—only blink and see up and down, unable to move any part of your body. Hence, locked-in. Scary stuff, I tell you!

Attitude

As a survivor, every second of every day, you have to approach every day as if you were going to move forward in any way you can. I know this sounds like something you have heard before; I am here to let you know you can do it. We all have bad days; it's how you respond that makes you go to the next level. I caught it with the tinnitus and vertigo on a daily basis.

As a survivor, you have to have tremendous faith in all you do. This has been my big factor in my recovery. We all have challenging days, and personally I find those days are what I called "game-changer days." These are the ones that you decide to forge ahead, and when you do, the progress you make those days are amazing.

I'm starting to notice that people talk an awful lot about what they are going to do—complain. It is the few that do something about it! I was blessed to start my PT, or shall I say, begin to move. My wife had to battle with insurance, as most had written me off and had no problem putting a forty-nine-year-old in a rest home. Praise God I have a wife that fought for me every single step.

After coming out of my coma, I was moved to a new hospital, where Chip introduced me to sitting up. I was what I called a "weeble-wobble." I could not hold my head up. I literally would fall over and could not control it.

What is this? I kept saying in my mind. *Why am I doing this?* I really thought, after all this, I would be able to go back to the way I was quickly. I had my butt handed to me no doubt in looking back at the photos. Wrong, so wrong I was. So after failing many, many times to sit up, Chip kept me motivated to keep trying, so I did find myself having to look at this as a challenge that I was going to take head on. *No time to feel sorry for myself. Let's get to work,* I told Chip (in my mind I told him and tried to write it down). A fist bump, and we were off.

After concurring sitting, I had to learn to kick my legs and try and get my left leg to keep up with my right leg. I actually, to this day, still cannot tie my shoes, walk without assistance, or attempt and look like a drunken sailor, let alone sometimes forget I have a left arm and leg. These are just a few things survivors deal with; it's up to us how we respond! I literally would try and do an exercise and have to take a nap. The mind is so powerful; you can fill it with negativity or saturate it with positive thoughts.

Take the time to write down ten things you are thankful for. If you can't write yet, you can ask a partner to write it down! Review this every day no matter what. You will have bad days guaranteed, so when you feel defeated, read this or have someone read it to you. I have no doubt that this will help you. The people that are around you daily can see your struggles. I'm not that good at talking about struggles, but your caregiver, who has seen firsthand, will be sure to be your voice.

Try not to be discouraged when your story is being told, and the person quickly turns to how it would affect them. I have many times been asked question like, "I once thought I was having a stroke. My relative had a stroke, and he or she is fine. Why are you not?" or "I had chest pains the other day. Do you think I was having a stroke?" Really! People in general are self-centered and think of themselves first in most cases. If you see someone that is a survivor that is out in public, please take the time to show a little empathy and try and talk with their caregiver to give words of encouragement. You just never know how a smile or a positive word may be a huge deal to them. This goes for anyone, really—a positive or loving comment can have a huge impact.

I would rather be disabled and have a good attitude than to not be and have a bad attitude! The brain takes eighteen years to grow and a lifetime to mature. In other words, it matures through time, which means no matter how old you are, your brain is maturing. Now do we put positive in while it is maturing or negative? That is up to you. As for me, what little space I have left in my brain, I choose positive thoughts.

FAST
Face, Arm, Speech, Time.

I say all this because in talking to people in my stroke support group, there are many of us that are misdiagnosed, and what's even more scary is our youth are a great danger here. Did you know there is a pediatric stroke? It is a myth that stroke affects only the elderly. Twenty-five to a hundred thousand newborns have a stroke. According to the UNICEF website, 130 million babies are born each year that are registered. This figure, I'm sure, is higher. Taking that number alone means 32,500 newborns a year have a stroke.

Patients who arrive within three hours of their first symptoms and receive proper care often have less disability three months after stroke than those who received delayed care. Stroke is the fifth-leading cause of death in the United States and number one in disability. Every four minutes, someone dies of stroke. Every forty seconds, someone has a stroke in the US alone. One to six deaths from cardiovascular disease was due to stroke. Stroke is the leading cause of disability per the American Heart Association.

I arrived via ambulance to the hospital within thirteen minutes of my symptoms. I did not receive proper care. The FAST acronym recommended by the American Heart Association was not used for my diagnosis. FAST saves lives and may save you or your loved one too.

Confidence

Confidence comes from knowing Christ. As I lie in a hospital bed, I could hear conversations about me being a vegetable and all conversations about me, negative or positive. I just wanted to scream! In my mind, as I open my eyes, I realized that was all I could do. I am trapped, and there's nothing I can do. The only movement is blinking. I would try over and over to move a finger or a toe—I was trapped, and it may be forever. Am I dead?

Please know, anyone reading this, that your loved one can hear you while in a coma. Do not listen to what anyone tells you. I'm telling you from firsthand experience that we hear everything. The "I love you's" kept me going. They will keep your loved ones encouraged. There is nothing wrong with pulling a chair close, reading scripture, and praying in their ear. This resonates and gives hope.

If it were not for my wife, Misty, I would not be here. She advocated for me constantly; I knew it and could hear it. Some of the people were rude to her, and I just wanted to sit up and defend her. Every one of the hospital staff had given up on me.

Locked-in syndrome affects one percent of stroke patients. I was a one-percent what? It is a condition that there is no treatment or cure. And extremely rare for patients to recover any significant motor function. About ninety percent die within the first four months if it's onset. My wife was told to get a book called *The Diving-Bell and the Butterfly*, to read it, and to accept this was now me. I felt the most vulnerable I had ever been in my life—lonely and afraid that I would get a mean person on one of the shifts. I was asking God, "Why have I come so far to now be here?" You want to talk about taking time for him, I was all ears—or in my case, ear. From what I had just gone through, I now was a one hundred percent so I had that to go fight this battle. It was God that said, *I have got it from here*. He got me this far, so who was I to have a shred of doubt. I had hope through my lord, Jesus Christ.

Looking back, the only way to look is up. And you talk about crying out to Jesus; I was crying alright. I found myself going back to my youth, a childlike faith that is a beautiful thing. My dad was and still is my hero on Earth. I always felt safe when he was near, but now my heavenly Father gave me great comfort. As an adult, pre-stroke, I had a tremendous amount of confidence, and now I find myself in the position of humility beyond my comprehension.

I was on a journey not knowing where I was going. God was driving us on this journey, showing me a clip of my life. It seemed He was proud of me? I'm no one special; heck, I'm just a dumb average joe on this rollercoaster we call life. In His eyes, I was special, and guess what? You are too. I was locked into God, and this gave me a peace that in the flesh I simply could not handle. I was freaking out! *Keep your eyes on me*, He would say. His eyes were the most clear-blue eyes that I could see was love.

As I write this, I find emotions overflow as I go back to that moment. The feeling of being like a child again, looking toward his parents for guidance. I had the best guidance I could get and the best friend I could ever have. This was a terrifying journey, but one that I had no choice but to embrace it. My Lord and Savior was leading the way, and I was slowly coming to the end.

When I was finally able to move, my wife asked me if I saw Jesus, and I blinked to let her know I did. She would have to wait a month for me to be able to communicate the story. I was so excited to tell the story that I would attempt to write it down. I actually would get frustrated—it's simply not legible at all. My brain thought I was writing it down pretty well, but come to find out later, after seeing the notes the family kept, it was not legible at all.

> Once you have been confronted with a life-and-death situation, trivia no longer matters; your perspective grows and grows, and you live in a deeper level. There is no time for pettiness. (Margaretta Rockefeller)

God placed on my heart to have an attitude of gratitude, and as you rise in glory, you sink in pride.

I Will Never Be the Same

I will be forever changed. I have died of self and have a different thought process than I did. In my past, I was of the world and thought I was a follower of Christ, but now I live my life to be the most like him as I can—easier said than done, I tell you. Every person has a story and a reason for their actions, some good and some bad. I have a deeper understanding and find myself hovering like a drone overhead, seeing the big picture of people and truly believing there is good in all of us.

I know I'm being watched in everything I do, and not just by my heavenly Father. "How will He respond to this?," a question I can see many ask as I go through life on earth. You can tell in the back of some people's minds, *Will this change His course?* Sometimes I'm challenged, like all of us, and quickly stay on course, looking to bring as many as I can with me to return to heaven. I long for that peace I experienced that was unlike any peace I have ever experienced. I wanna go back, but I know that I have work to do here first.

When I first returned home I had an attitude that I wanted to back now—my timing. When he said I have big plans for you, I had to step back and think back to that moment in time where I was face-to-face with him. It has taken me almost five years to tell my story. Partly because I did not want the memories of all that happened to me to flood back. Watching some one hundred videos and looking at over eight hundred photos my wife took has caused many a sleepless night and a stirring in my heart to do what God has asked. Another reason is, I tried to write for years and simply could not put pen to paper. My brain was still scrambled and could not finish a thought process.

Thankful

Thankful for my wife, Misty; our kids; Mom and Dad; Brandi; Papa; Nick Maragos Marcus Rodriguez; Dr. Michael Lusk; Lois Grider; Drs. Brent and Amy Lovett; Janice Rosen; John; Kelly and Madison DeAngelis; Amanda Hope-Kibble; Sherry and Bobby Stein;

Brenda Fioretti; Jonathon Pentecost; Bro Pat; Chipster; and a lot of the staff at Landmark and Brookdale, to name a few. Support and love from these people, and more that I'm sure I've missed, had a huge impact on me. I will forever be grateful and humbled by your love, and the walk with you by my side is a true blessing. I feel rich in relationships and am looking forward to making more as I move forward.

The Fundraiser

It was a long time before my disability benefits started, and like most people that have been through a health crisis, you come home to being broke. The harsh reality is, many people don't plan on becoming disabled. As the main provider, it hits twice as hard because you feel even more useless. I couldn't even think straight, let alone work. I was home, but that darn reality kicked in hard.

Many of my friends decided to have a fundraiser for me. I was and still am so humbled by the amount of people who showed up that night to help us. Misty wheeled me into the restaurant, and there were so many people that I found myself overcome with emotion and I exhausted myself quickly. I wanted to speak to each and every person but simply could not do it. I did manage to muster up enough strength to stand out of my wheelchair while holding on to the table to give all the glory to my Lord and Savior, then bawling like a baby.

A part of me was so thankful that I could remember all my friends, and another part wished I could hug each and every one. I enjoyed sitting back in my wheelchair and just so humbly looking back on my life journey so far and watching everyone interact with one another. Taking the high road did pay off. I can say, without a doubt, I always tried to be fair and honest in my dealings with people. You see, I wasn't really on this life journey to make money; we need money to live, hence the fundraiser.

*****

I was always excited about the relationships I could and did form. My business was real estate, and I had been at it for more than half my life in Southwest Florida. My dad was in commercial real estate, and I chose residential—the passion for this type of real estate, for me, was the joy and excitement each day would bring. "Who would I meet today?" "Will I hear from any of my friends?" or "What is happening out there?" I would ask. The gift of being able to see what a piece of property could be fascinated me. I could visualize where my latest customers should live based on what was important to them.

This was and is a gift that has been passed through generations. If God asks me to get back in the game, so to speak, I would be there in a heartbeat. I keep hearing, *Be still,* and *Be thankful I can now communicate my story.* Like everything I do, I go full throttle and, as we say in my circle, go straight into the wave with no fear.

You see, I am one who would rather do something and fail than sit back and wonder. I would call it the "coulda, shoulda woulda's." I am so excited to share with you that, at times, when I go back like that Eddie Money song, "I Wanna Go Back," I wish I could do the things I could pre-stroke. I then snap back and am okay with where I am now.

I wish all people the best in everything, and know we all have a gift that God has given us. It's up to us to go find it. Go find it, and ask for his hand while searching. You and I were not built to do this life thing on our own. We are loving beings that need love and are built to be in relationships. After what I have been through, I have gained so much wisdom from it. I still have so far to go but am ready! Bitterness is a blessing blocker and one that hurts, so do yourself a favor and forgive while you can. Regret is a tough one, and yet one that can be avoided.

Thank you for taking the time to read my journey. I pray this will encourage you to stay strong while in a struggle. We all go through struggles. Let's face it: it's easy when things are going good, but it's when times get tough you find out who you are. With me, what you see is what you get. I always say, "I is who I is." I'm the same behind closed doors, as I am just talking to a stranger. My journey is a lot of pain, but there are many blessings along the way.

Let's not forget the mind is very powerful, and what you feed it becomes your belief. Personally, I believe God has a plan for everyone; now I have no doubt he does! I hope my personal stories of my life—that at times may be boring to you, but hang in there—is all connected. My life versus Hebrews 11:1, "Now faith is confidence in what we hope for and assurance about what we do not see." I hope you enjoy this glimpse into my journey, and my prayers are that at the end of this, your faith will be strengthened, inspired, and ready to take on life's journey in your own way.

> Once you have been confronted with a life-and-death situation, trivia no longer matters your perspective grows and you live in a deeper level. There's no time for pettiness. (Margaretta Rockefeller)

"Nothing Compares" by Third Day is a song that speaks to me. There is a part of the chorus, "I see all the people waiting all their time, building up their riches for a life that's fine." Absolutely nothing compares to Him. The peace and joy He can bring you is beyond anything you can even imagine. We think, *If I only had...* You fill in the blank and see for yourself: material things come and go, but His love for you and me is everlasting. If I had the gift of singing, I would sing to you and all that would listen. We won't go there, as my singing is one that causes people to run for the hills. Clearly not my gift, but I admire anyone that takes their gift to the highest level they can to glorify Him.

We as believers want that well-done. My good and faithful servant, as we enter heaven, I'm here to spread the word that it is an amazing place that I want all to go to. It brings comfort to me knowing where I'm going, which helps me to focus on my mission of others to join me there.

Tears of gratitude run down my face as I reflect on the blessings that have been given to me!

Positive thoughts. Attitude of gratitude.

Whatever you believe, you can achieve explanation every morning you were given the opportunity to improve and count your blessings. You rise in glory as you sink in pride. (Chris Adkins)

Scriptures I find helpful on faith:

That your faith might not rest in the wisdom of me but in the power of GOD. (1 Corinthians 2:5)

And whatever you ask in prayer, you will receive if you have faith. (Matthew 21:22)

For nothing will be impossible without God. (Luke 1:37)

For we walk by faith, not by sight. (2 Corinthians 5:7)

And without faith it is impossible to please God. Because anyone who comes to him must believe that he exists and that he rewards those who earnestly seek him. (Hebrews 11:6)

Yet we know that a person is not justified by works of the law but through faith in Jesus Christ, so we also have believed in Christ Jesus, in order to be justified by faith in Christ and not by works of the law, because by works of the law no one will be justified. (Galatians 2:16)

And Jesus answered them, "Have faith in God. Truly, I say to you, whoever says to this mountain, be taken up and thrown into the sea and does not doubt in his heart, but believes that we he says will come to pass, it will be done for him. Therefore I tell you, whatever you ask in prayer, believe that you have received it, and it will be yours." (Mark 11:22–24)

For nothing will be impossible with God. (Luke 1:37)

If you need wisdom, ask our generous God, and He will give it to you. He will not rebuke you for asking. But when you ask Him, be sure that your faith is in God alone... Do not waiver, for a person with divided loyalty is as unsettled as a wave of the sea that is blown and tossed by the wind. (James 1:5–6)

About the Author

Chris Adkins a real estate professional for three decades in Southwest Florida, totaling over $400 million in volume. Chris is also known for his accomplishments in the powerlifting arena. A top ten cross country runner in the state of Florida to transforming his body from a runner to lifter. Chris lives with his wife, Misty, in Utah, where he enjoys time with his three grown children.

CPSIA information can be obtained
at www.ICGtesting.com
Printed in the USA
LVHW011038221121
704099LV00009B/219

9 781638 748786